JUICE YOUR LIBIDO

Boosting Sexual Performance Naturally through Juicing

ANN E. WILLIAMS

TABLE OF CONTENTS

Introduction

Dear Reader,

Welcome to JUICE YOUR LIBIDO, a comprehensive guide to enhancing your sexual performance and vitality through the power of juicing. In this book, we embark on a journey to explore how nature's bounty of fruits, vegetables, and herbs can revitalize your libido, increase stamina, and improve overall sexual health.

Today, many individuals struggle with stress, fatigue, and the demands of daily life, which can take a toll on their sexual well-being. Instead of resorting to synthetic supplements or invasive treatments, JUICE YOUR LIBIDO offers a holistic approach to revitalizing your sexual health naturally.

Throughout this book, you will discover a wealth of information on the benefits of juicing for sexual performance, including:

- Understanding the connection between nutrition and sexual health: Learn how the foods you consume can impact your libido, hormone levels, and overall sexual function.

- Exploring the science behind juicing: Delve into the nutritional properties of fruits, vegetables, and herbs that can enhance sexual desire, arousal, and performance.

- Creating delicious and nutritious juice recipes: Unlock the potential of nature's aphrodisiacs with a collection of mouthwatering juice blends designed to boost libido, increase energy, and support sexual vitality.

- Incorporating juicing into your lifestyle: Discover practical tips and strategies for incorporating juicing into your daily routine, from selecting the best ingredients to maximizing the benefits of your juices.

- Addressing common sexual health concerns: Gain insight into natural remedies for erectile dysfunction, low libido, and other issues that can affect sexual performance, supported by scientific research and expert advice.

- Embracing a holistic approach to sexual wellness: Learn how to nourish your body, mind, and spirit to create a balanced and fulfilling sexual experience, both individually and with a partner.

Whether you are seeking to reignite the spark in your relationship, overcome sexual health challenges, or simply optimize your overall well-being, JUICE YOUR LIBIDO provides you with the tools and knowledge to transform your sexual health naturally.

I invite you to embark on this journey with an open mind and a willingness to explore the transformative power of juicing. Together, let us unlock the secrets to a vibrant and fulfilling sex life, one delicious sip at a time.

Here's to juicing your libido and reclaiming your sexual vitality!

With warm regards.

Understanding the Power of Juicing for Sexual Health

Maintaining optimal sexual health can sometimes feel like an elusive goal. However, the solution to enhancing sexual well-being may be simpler than you think: juicing. Juicing, the process of extracting liquid from fruits and vegetables, has gained popularity for its numerous health benefits, including its potential to boost sexual health. This comprehensive note explores the power of juicing as a natural and effective way to support sexual vitality and wellness.

1. Nutrient-Rich Ingredients:
Juicing provides a convenient and efficient way to consume a wide variety of nutrients essential for sexual health. Fruits and vegetables such as spinach, kale, beets, carrots, berries, and citrus fruits are rich sources of vitamins, minerals, antioxidants, and phytochemicals that promote circulation, hormone balance, and overall well-being.

2. Blood Flow and Circulation:
A key factor in sexual function is adequate blood flow to the genital area. Certain fruits and vegetables, particularly those high in nitrates like beets and leafy greens, have been shown to improve blood flow and vasodilation, which may enhance arousal and sexual response.

3. Hormonal Balance:

Imbalances in hormones, such as testosterone and estrogen, can impact libido and sexual function. Juicing with ingredients like celery, broccoli, and watermelon may help support hormonal balance by providing essential nutrients and phytochemicals that regulate hormone production and metabolism.

4. Antioxidant Protection:
Oxidative stress caused by free radicals can damage cells and tissues throughout the body, including those involved in sexual function. Juicing with antioxidant-rich fruits and vegetables, such as blueberries, strawberries, and leafy greens, can help combat oxidative stress and protect against age-related decline in sexual health.

5. Detoxification and Cleansing:
Toxins and pollutants from environmental sources can accumulate in the body and interfere with sexual health. Juicing with detoxifying ingredients like ginger, lemon,

and cilantro can support the body's natural detoxification processes, promoting overall health and vitality.

6. Energy and Stamina:
Fatigue and low energy levels can diminish sexual desire and performance. Juicing with nutrient-dense ingredients provides a natural source of energy and stamina, supporting physical endurance and vitality for enhanced sexual experiences.

7. Mental and Emotional Well-Being:
Stress, anxiety, and depression can negatively impact sexual desire and satisfaction. Juicing with mood-boosting ingredients like bananas, avocados, and dark leafy greens can help regulate neurotransmitters and promote feelings of relaxation, happiness, and emotional connection.

8. Hydration and Lubrication:

Proper hydration is essential for maintaining healthy mucous membranes and lubrication during sexual activity. Juicing with hydrating fruits and vegetables, such as cucumbers, watermelon, and oranges, can support hydration levels and promote natural lubrication for improved comfort and pleasure.

9. Digestive Health:
A healthy digestive system is crucial for nutrient absorption and overall well-being, including sexual health. Juicing with fiber-rich ingredients like apples, carrots, and spinach can support digestive health and regularity, reducing bloating and discomfort that may interfere with sexual enjoyment.

10. Lifestyle Support:
In addition to juicing, adopting a holistic approach to sexual health that includes regular exercise, stress management, adequate sleep, and healthy relationships is

essential for overall well-being. Juicing can complement these lifestyle factors by providing a convenient and enjoyable way to nourish the body and support sexual vitality.

Juicing offers a natural and effective strategy for enhancing sexual health and wellness. By incorporating nutrient-rich fruits and vegetables into your daily diet, you can support circulation, hormone balance, energy levels, and overall vitality for a fulfilling and satisfying sex life. So, raise a glass to juicing for sexual health and reap the benefits of nature's potent elixirs.

Chapter 1: The Science Behind Libido and Nutrition

Exploring the Relationship Between Diet and Sexual Health

In today's world, where the pursuit of optimal health encompasses every aspect of our lives, the connection between nutrition and sexual health is gaining increasing attention. This note delves into the intricate relationship between diet and libido, shedding light on the scientific underpinnings that influence our sexual vitality.

Understanding Libido:
At the heart of the discussion lies libido, often referred to as sexual desire or drive. Libido is a complex interplay of physiological, psychological, and social factors that contribute to our sexual arousal and motivation. While libido can vary

greatly among individuals and can be influenced by age, hormonal balance, stress levels, and relationship dynamics, emerging research suggests that nutrition plays a significant role in modulating this essential aspect of human sexuality.

Nutrition and Sexual Health:
Nutrition serves as the fuel that powers our bodies, influencing everything from energy levels to hormonal balance. When it comes to sexual health, certain nutrients have been found to have a profound impact on libido, sexual function, and overall sexual satisfaction.

Key Nutrients for Sexual Health:
1. Omega-3 Fatty Acids: Found in fatty fish like salmon, as well as flaxseeds and walnuts, omega-3 fatty acids support cardiovascular health and circulation, crucial factors in achieving and maintaining arousal.

2. Antioxidants: Foods rich in antioxidants, such as fruits, vegetables, and dark chocolate, help combat oxidative stress and inflammation, which can impede blood flow and contribute to erectile dysfunction or decreased sexual desire.

3. Zinc: Essential for testosterone production and sperm health, zinc-rich foods like oysters, beef, and pumpkin seeds play a vital role in maintaining healthy libido and sexual function.

4. B Vitamins: B vitamins, particularly B6, B9 (folate), and B12, are involved in neurotransmitter synthesis and hormone regulation, influencing mood, energy levels, and sexual desire. Sources include leafy greens, legumes, eggs, and lean meats.

5. L-arginine: An amino acid that promotes vasodilation and blood flow to the genitals, l-arginine-rich foods like poultry, dairy, nuts, and seeds may enhance sexual performance and satisfaction.

Dietary Patterns and Sexual Health:

In addition to individual nutrients, dietary patterns such as the Mediterranean diet and the DASH (Dietary Approaches to Stop Hypertension) diet have been associated with improved sexual function and libido. These diets emphasize whole foods, lean proteins, fruits, vegetables, and healthy fats while limiting processed foods, sugar, and unhealthy fats, supporting overall cardiovascular health and circulation—a cornerstone of sexual vitality.

Beyond Nutrition: Lifestyle Factors Impacting Libido:
While nutrition plays a pivotal role in sexual health, it is essential to recognize that other lifestyle factors, including exercise, stress management, sleep quality, and relationship dynamics, also influence libido and sexual function. By adopting a holistic approach to health and well-being, addressing both nutritional and lifestyle factors, individuals can optimize their sexual health and vitality,

fostering a fulfilling and satisfying intimate life.

As our understanding of the intricate interplay between nutrition and sexual health continues to evolve, empowering individuals with knowledge and resources to make informed dietary choices becomes paramount. By prioritizing nutrient-rich foods, adopting healthy lifestyle habits, and seeking support when needed, individuals can harness the power of nutrition to enhance their libido, revitalize their sexual health, and reclaim a fulfilling and satisfying intimate life.

Nutrients That Fuel Your Libido

Understanding the intricate relationship between nutrition and libido is crucial for optimizing sexual health and vitality. This note delves into the science behind libido and highlights key nutrients that play a significant role in fueling sexual desire and function.

Libido, often referred to as sexual desire or drive, is a complex interplay of physiological, psychological, and environmental factors. While factors such as stress, hormones, and relationship dynamics influence libido, nutrition also plays a pivotal role in supporting sexual health and function.

The Role of Nutrients in Libido

Nutrients act as building blocks for various physiological processes in the body, including those related to sexual function. Certain vitamins, minerals, and other compounds have been shown to have a direct impact on libido by supporting hormone production, enhancing blood flow, and promoting overall sexual health.

Key Nutrients for Libido

1. Zinc: This mineral plays a crucial role in testosterone production, a hormone essential for maintaining sexual desire and function in both men and women. Foods rich in zinc include oysters, beef, pumpkin seeds, and chickpeas.
2. Vitamin D: Low levels of vitamin D have been linked to decreased libido and sexual dysfunction. Sunlight exposure and fortified foods such as fatty fish, eggs, and fortified dairy products are excellent sources of vitamin D.
3. Omega-3 Fatty Acids: These healthy fats support cardiovascular health and enhance blood flow, which is essential for sexual arousal and function. Sources of omega-3 fatty acids include fatty fish (salmon, mackerel, sardines), flaxseeds, chia seeds, and walnuts.

4. Vitamin C: This antioxidant vitamin helps improve blood circulation and supports the health of blood vessels, which are critical for sexual arousal and performance. Citrus fruits, berries, kiwi, and bell peppers are excellent sources of vitamin C.

5. Magnesium: Magnesium plays a role in neurotransmitter function and muscle relaxation, both of which are important for sexual function. Foods rich in magnesium include leafy greens, nuts, seeds, whole grains, and legumes.

6. L-arginine: This amino acid is a precursor to nitric oxide, a molecule that helps relax blood vessels and improve blood flow to the genitals, thereby enhancing arousal and performance. L-arginine-rich foods include red meat, poultry, fish, dairy products, and nuts.

7. B Vitamins: B vitamins, particularly B6, B9 (folate), and B12, are involved in hormone regulation and neurotransmitter synthesis, which are important for sexual health. Foods rich in B vitamins include

whole grains, leafy greens, legumes, eggs, and lean meats.

8. Iron: Iron deficiency can lead to fatigue and decreased energy levels, which may negatively impact libido. Red meat, poultry, fish, beans, lentils, and fortified cereals are good sources of iron.

Incorporating Libido-Boosting Foods into Your Diet

To optimize libido and sexual health, aim to incorporate a variety of nutrient-rich foods into your diet. Focus on whole foods such as fruits, vegetables, lean proteins, whole grains, nuts, seeds, and healthy fats. Additionally, maintaining a balanced diet, staying hydrated, and limiting processed foods and excess sugar can further support sexual wellness.

By understanding the science behind libido and nutrition and incorporating libido-boosting nutrients into your diet, you can support sexual health and vitality. Remember that individual needs may vary, so it's essential to listen to your body and consult with a healthcare professional for personalized guidance. With a holistic approach to nutrition and lifestyle, you can fuel your libido and reclaim your sexual wellness.

How Juicing Can Enhance Sexual Performance

In the pursuit of a fulfilling and vibrant sex life, many factors come into play, including lifestyle, mindset, and yes, nutrition. The relationship between diet and sexual health has been an area of interest for researchers and health enthusiasts alike, with studies uncovering the intricate connections between certain nutrients and libido. This note delves into the science behind libido and nutrition, exploring how juicing can play a role in enhancing sexual performance.

The Role of Nutrition in Sexual Health

Nutrition plays a crucial role in supporting overall health and well-being, and its effects extend to sexual health as well. Certain nutrients have been found to have specific benefits for libido and sexual function, including:

1. Zinc: This essential mineral is involved in the production of testosterone, a key hormone in regulating sexual desire and performance. Zinc deficiency has been linked to decreased libido and sexual dysfunction in both men and women.

2. Vitamins C and E: These antioxidants help protect against oxidative stress and

inflammation, which can negatively impact sexual health. Vitamin C is also involved in the synthesis of collagen, which supports the health of blood vessels and erectile function.

3. Omega-3 fatty acids: Found in fatty fish, flaxseeds, and walnuts, omega-3 fatty acids have anti-inflammatory properties and may improve blood flow, which is essential for erectile function and sexual arousal.

4. Arginine: This amino acid is a precursor to nitric oxide, a molecule that helps relax blood vessels and improve circulation. Increasing arginine intake may enhance erectile function and sexual satisfaction.

5. Phytonutrients: Found in colorful fruits and vegetables, phytonutrients have antioxidant and anti-inflammatory properties that support overall health and may positively impact sexual function.

The Benefits of Juicing for Sexual Performance

Juicing, the process of extracting juice from fruits and vegetables, offers a convenient and efficient way to consume a wide variety of nutrients that support sexual health. Here's how juicing can enhance sexual performance:

1. Nutrient Density: Juicing allows for the consumption of large quantities of fruits and vegetables in a concentrated form, providing a potent dose of vitamins, minerals, and phytonutrients that support overall health, including sexual function.

2. Hydration: Proper hydration is essential for optimal sexual health, as it helps maintain blood flow and lubrication. Juicing provides a hydrating source of fluids, along with essential electrolytes that support hydration and overall well-being.

3. Digestive Health: Many fruits and vegetables used in juicing are rich in fiber, which supports digestive health and may indirectly benefit sexual function by promoting nutrient absorption and eliminating toxins from the body.

4. Alkalizing Properties: Some fruits and vegetables, such as leafy greens and citrus fruits, have alkalizing properties that help balance pH levels in the body. An alkaline environment may support hormonal balance and overall vitality, which are important factors in sexual health.

5. Variety and Flavor: Juicing allows for creativity and variety in the selection of ingredients, making it easy to incorporate a diverse range of nutrients into the diet. Additionally, the natural sweetness of fruits can enhance the flavor of juices, making them a delicious and enjoyable addition to daily nutrition.

Incorporating juicing into a balanced and nutritious diet can be a simple yet effective way to support sexual health and enhance sexual performance. By providing a concentrated source of vitamins, minerals, and phytonutrients, juicing nourishes the body and promotes overall vitality, contributing to a fulfilling and satisfying sex life. However, it's important to remember that while juicing can complement a healthy lifestyle, it is not a substitute for medical treatment or professional advice. As with any dietary changes, it's advisable to consult with a healthcare provider or nutritionist to ensure that juicing is appropriate for individual needs and goals. With mindful nutrition and lifestyle choices, individuals can empower themselves to optimize their sexual health and experience the pleasures of intimacy to the fullest.

Chapter 2: Juicing Essentials

Getting Started: Choosing the Right Juicer and Ingredients

Juicing has become increasingly popular as more people seek to incorporate healthy habits into their daily routines. Whether you're a seasoned juicer or just starting out on your journey to better health, understanding the essentials of juicing is crucial for success. In this comprehensive guide, we'll explore everything you need to know to get started with juicing, from selecting the right juicer to choosing the best ingredients for optimal nutrition and flavor.

Understanding the Benefits of Juicing

Before delving into the practical aspects of juicing, it's important to understand the myriad benefits it offers. Juicing allows you to easily consume a variety of fruits and vegetables in concentrated form, providing a potent dose of vitamins, minerals, and antioxidants. By extracting the juice from produce, you can enjoy increased energy, improved digestion, clearer skin, and enhanced immune function. Additionally, juicing can be a convenient way to increase your intake of fruits and vegetables, especially for those who struggle to meet recommended daily servings.

Choosing the Right Juicer

One of the first decisions you'll need to make when starting your juicing journey is selecting the right juicer for your needs. There are several types of juicers available, each with its own unique features and benefits. Centrifugal juicers are popular for their speed and efficiency, making them ideal for beginners and those short on time.

Masticating juicers, on the other hand, operate at lower speeds and produce juice with higher nutrient content and longer shelf life. Twin gear juicers offer the highest level of juice extraction and are well-suited for serious juicing enthusiasts. Consider factors such as price, ease of use, and maintenance requirements when choosing a juicer that aligns with your preferences and lifestyle.

Exploring Juicing Ingredients
Once you've selected your juicer, it's time to explore the wide array of ingredients available for juicing. Fruits such as apples, oranges, and berries add sweetness and flavor to your juices, while vegetables like spinach, kale, and cucumbers provide essential vitamins and minerals.

Experiment with different combinations of fruits and vegetables to find flavor profiles that appeal to your taste buds. Don't be afraid to get creative and incorporate herbs, spices, and superfoods like ginger, turmeric, and chia seeds for added health benefits.

Remember to choose organic produce whenever possible to minimize exposure to pesticides and chemicals.

Tips for Juicing Success

To ensure a successful juicing experience, there are a few tips to keep in mind. Start by thoroughly washing and preparing your fruits and vegetables, removing any stems, seeds, or tough skins. Experiment with different produce combinations to find your favorite flavors and nutrient profiles.

Drink your fresh juice immediately to maximize nutritional content and prevent oxidation. If you're unable to consume your juice right away, store it in an airtight container in the refrigerator for up to 24 hours. And finally, clean your juicer thoroughly after each use to prevent bacteria buildup and maintain optimal performance.

Juicing is a simple yet powerful way to boost your health and vitality, providing a convenient means of consuming a wide variety of fruits and vegetables. By choosing the right juicer and ingredients, you can create delicious and nutritious concoctions that support your overall well-being. Whether you're looking to kickstart a healthy lifestyle or simply enjoy the refreshing taste of fresh juice, juicing essentials will guide you on your journey to vibrant health and vitality.

Juicing Techniques and Tips for Maximum Nutrient Retention

Juicing has become a popular way to consume a variety of fruits and vegetables, ensuring you get a healthy dose of vitamins, minerals, and antioxidants in an easily digestible form. The technique of juicing involves extracting the liquid content from fresh fruits and vegetables, leaving behind the pulp. While juicing can be a beneficial addition to your diet, the method of extraction and the handling of ingredients play crucial roles in the nutritional outcome of the juice. This note covers essential juicing techniques and tips designed to maximize nutrient retention.

- Understanding Juicing

1. Types of Juicers:
   - Centrifugal Juicers: These juicers shred ingredients with a rapidly spinning disk to extract juice. While quick and cost-effective, they tend to generate heat and expose ingredients to air, which can reduce nutrient levels.
   - Masticating Juicers (Cold Press): These operate at slower speeds and crush fruits and vegetables against a screen, minimizing

heat and oxidation. This method preserves more enzymes and nutrients.

- Triturating Juicers: These use twin gears to crush and press produce at even slower speeds than masticating juicers, offering the highest yield and nutrient retention.

- Hydraulic Press Juicers: These extract juice by pressing the fruit or vegetable pulp under high pressure, producing the highest quality juice in terms of nutrient density and yield.

- Maximizing Nutrient Retention

2. Handling and Preparation of Ingredients:
- Freshness Matters: Use fresh, organic produce to avoid pesticides and chemicals. Fresh vegetables and fruits retain more nutrients.
- Proper Storage: Store produce in a cool, dark place or in refrigerated conditions to slow nutrient degradation.
- Pre-Juicing Preparation: Wash all produce thoroughly. Peeling should be

avoided where possible, as many nutrients and fibers are found in the skins.

3. Juicing Techniques:
   - Slow Juicing: Use a slow juicer if possible. The slower speed reduces heat and air exposure, preserving enzymes and preventing oxidation.
   - Pulsing vs. Steady Juicing: Pulsing can sometimes help in reducing the temperature buildup during juicing.

4. Timing of Juicing:
   - Immediate Consumption: Drink juice immediately after preparation to benefit from the maximum nutrient content. Delaying consumption can lead to nutrient loss through oxidation.

5. Juice Combinations:
   - Balancing Ingredients: Combining a variety of fruits and vegetables can help in balancing nutrients and enhancing absorption. For example, adding a vitamin

C-rich fruit like orange to green leafy vegetable juices can enhance iron absorption from the greens.
 - Adding Fats: Incorporating a small amount of healthy fat, such as flaxseed oil or a slice of avocado, can increase the bioavailability of fat-soluble vitamins.

- Other Considerations

6. Temperature and Storage:
 - Keep It Cool: Always juice at cool temperatures if possible, and store any leftover juice in airtight containers filled to the brim to minimize air exposure, in the refrigerator for up to 24 hours.

7. Cleaning Your Juicer:
 - Immediate Cleaning: Clean your juicer immediately after use to prevent pulp and residue from drying, which makes it harder to clean and can harbor bacteria.

8. Nutrient Dense Juicing:

- Leafy Greens: Incorporate leafy greens like spinach, kale, and Swiss chard, which are high in vitamins A, C, and K, as well as minerals like iron and calcium.
- Herbs and Spices: Adding ingredients like parsley, cilantro, turmeric, or ginger can boost the antioxidant content and flavor profile of your juices.

Juicing, when done correctly, can be a fantastic way to supplement your diet with high-quality nutrients. By choosing the right type of juicer, handling ingredients properly, and consuming juice immediately, you can ensure that you receive the maximum health benefits from your juicing efforts. Remember, while juicing is beneficial, it should complement a balanced diet rich in whole foods to ensure you receive adequate dietary fiber and other essential nutrients.

Incorporating Juicing into Your Daily Routine

Juicing is a popular health trend that involves extracting the nourishing liquids from fresh fruits and vegetables. It can be a powerful way to boost your intake of vitamins, minerals, and antioxidants, and when incorporated thoughtfully into your daily routine, can support a variety of health benefits. Whether you're looking to enhance your energy, improve digestion, or just boost your daily intake of nutrients, understanding the essentials of juicing can help you start on the right foot.

Why Juice?
Juicing allows you to consume an optimal amount of vegetables in an efficient manner. Some find they can more easily meet their daily target for vegetables by drinking them instead of eating them whole. Juicing can also help the body absorb nutrients better as it breaks down vegetables and fruits, bypassing what can sometimes be a taxed

digestive system. Moreover, juicing can be a fun and tasty way to experiment with flavors and discover new ways to enjoy fresh produce.

Choosing the Right Juicer
There are several types of juicers on the market, including centrifugal, masticating, and triturating juicers, each having their own pros and cons. Centrifugal juicers are popular due to their speed and affordability, but they can be noisy and less efficient at extracting juice from leafy greens or wheatgrass. Masticating juicers operate at a slower speed, which helps to preserve nutrients and enzymes and can handle a wider variety of vegetables, including greens and herbs. Triturating juicers are the most efficient and also the most expensive, ideal for those who are very serious about juicing.

Understanding What to Juice
Almost any fruit and vegetable can be juiced, but some are more beneficial than

others. Leafy greens like spinach, kale, and Swiss chard are packed with chlorophyll and key vitamins that are easily absorbed in juice form. Carrots, beets, apples, and cucumbers are also excellent for juicing, providing essential nutrients and making for a palatable introduction for juicing newcomers. However, it's important to note that fruit juice should be consumed in moderation due to its high sugar content.

Incorporating Juicing into Your Routine Start your day with a glass of juice as a morning ritual to hydrate and energize yourself after hours of fasting overnight. This can also prevent the temptation to consume overly sugary beverages for breakfast. Alternatively, drinking juice before a meal can serve as a great appetizer, helping you to feel fuller and thus reducing the overall calorie intake.

Juice Combinations

Experiment with different combinations to maximize health benefits. For example, a juice blend of ginger, lemon, and beetroot can be a powerful detoxifier, while cucumber, apple, and spinach may serve as an invigorating energy booster. Understanding the properties of each ingredient can help you tailor your juices to your health needs.

Safety and Storage
Fresh juice is best consumed immediately after it is pressed since it can quickly lose its nutritional value. If storing juice, keep it in a tightly sealed container and consume within 24 hours to minimize nutrient loss. Always wash and, where necessary, peel fruits and vegetables to remove pesticides and contaminants before juicing.

Balancing Juicing with Whole Foods
While juicing can be a valuable addition to your diet, it should not replace whole foods, especially since juice lacks fiber, which is

crucial for healthy digestion. Ensure that your diet remains varied and balanced, including whole fruits and vegetables, grains, proteins, and fats.

Juicing offers an excellent avenue to boost nutrient intake and can be a delightful part of your daily health regimen. By understanding how to select a juicer, which produce to choose, and how to safely prepare and store juice, you can enjoy all the benefits that juicing has to offer while maintaining a balanced diet. Whether you're a seasoned juicer or just starting out, the key is to have fun and enjoy the vibrant flavors nature provides.

Chapter 3: Supercharged Juices for Libido

Aphrodisiac Ingredients: A Guide to Libido-Boosting Fruits, Vegetables, and Herbs

Supercharged Juices for Libido: Aphrodisiac Ingredients is a comprehensive guide designed to help individuals boost their libido through the power of natural juices. This guide dives into the world of aphrodisiac fruits, vegetables, and herbs, explaining their benefits and how they can be used to create potent, libido-enhancing beverages. The book is not just a recipe collection but also an educational resource on enhancing sexual health and overall vitality through diet.

- Key Concepts Explained:

1. Understanding Libido:

The book begins with an exploration of what libido is and how it is influenced by various factors including hormones, stress, sleep, and overall health. It sets the groundwork for understanding why certain foods have an impact on sexual desire and performance.

2. The Role of Nutrition in Sexual Health: There is a detailed discussion on how nutrition plays a critical role in sexual health. It covers how nutrients affect hormonal balance, blood flow, and energy levels, all of which are crucial for a healthy libido.

- Detailed Look at Aphrodisiac Ingredients:

3. Fruits:
- Watermelon: Rich in citrulline, which helps increase blood flow to sexual organs.
- Avocado: Loaded with potassium and vitamin E, enhancing energy and stamina.

- Bananas: High in potassium and B vitamins, essential for hormone production.
- Figs: Celebrated for their shape and texture, figs are high in amino acids that can increase libido.

4. Vegetables:
- Celery: Contains androstenone and androstenol, pheromones that can increase sexual arousal.
- Spinach: High in magnesium, which can help dilate blood vessels for better blood flow.
- Beets: Known for their ability to boost nitric oxide production and improve circulation.

5. Herbs:
- Ginseng: A powerful root known to enhance erectile function and sexual desire.
- Maca: Often referred to as Peruvian Viagra, it helps balance hormones and increase stamina.

- Ginkgo Biloba: Improves circulation and is thought to enhance sexual function by stimulating blood flow.

- Recipes and Juice Combinations:

6. Juice Recipes:
The book provides a variety of recipes that combine these aphrodisiac ingredients into delicious and potent juices. Each recipe includes detailed instructions and nutritional information, explaining how each ingredient contributes to increasing libido.

7. How to Incorporate These Juices into Your Daily Routine:
Practical advice on integrating these juices into daily meals, either as a morning tonic, an afternoon energizer, or an intimate prelude to an evening.

- Health Considerations:

8. Safety and Allergies:
Important cautions and potential side effects related to specific ingredients are discussed. The book advises consulting with a healthcare provider before starting any new diet, especially for those with underlying health conditions or who are taking medications.

9. Balancing Libido-Boosting Juices with a Healthy Lifestyle:
Emphasizes that while these juices can aid sexual health, they are most effective when used in conjunction with a balanced diet, regular exercise, and adequate sleep.

Supercharged Juices for Libido: Aphrodisiac Ingredients aims not only to enhance sexual vitality through specific foods but also to encourage a holistic approach to health and wellness. It is an essential guide for anyone looking to naturally enhance their libido and improve their sexual health through the power of juicing.

Recipes for Energy-Boosting Juices

Today, maintaining energy levels and a healthy libido can often seem challenging. Diet plays a crucial role in enhancing both, and incorporating specific, nutrient-dense juices into your daily routine can be a powerful way to boost your vitality and sexual health. This guide explores various energy-boosting juice recipes that are specifically designed to enhance libido and overall well-being.

The Role of Nutrition in Libido
Libido, or sexual desire, can be influenced by a variety of factors, including hormone levels, stress, sleep quality, and overall

health. Nutrients play a direct role in all these areas. For instance, certain vitamins and minerals can boost testosterone and estrogen levels, improve blood flow, and enhance mood, all of which can increase libido.

Key Nutrients for Enhancing Libido
- Vitamin C: Enhances blood circulation and increases arousal. Found in oranges, strawberries, and kiwi.
- Zinc: Boosts testosterone production, essential for both male and female libido. Rich sources include spinach, garlic, and pumpkin seeds.
- Magnesium: Reduces stress and anxiety, thereby potentially increasing libido. Available in leafy greens like spinach and Swiss chard.
- Potassium: Aids in hormone balance and energy levels. Bananas and avocados are great sources.
- Antioxidants: Combat oxidative stress and support vascular health, which is crucial for

sexual function. Berries, pomegranates, and beets are excellent choices.

Supercharged Juice Recipes
Here are several recipes designed to enhance energy and libido:

1. Tropical Desire
   - 1 cup fresh pineapple
   - 1 orange, peeled
   - 1/2 banana
   - 1/2 inch ginger root
   - Optional: A pinch of cayenne pepper for an extra kick

 This juice is packed with Vitamin C from orange and pineapple, enhancing blood flow and mood. Ginger adds a zesty flavor and stimulates circulation.

2. Berry Bliss
   - 1 cup mixed berries (strawberries, blueberries, raspberries)
   - 1 small beet, peeled and sliced

- 1/2 apple for sweetness

Berries and beets are rich in antioxidants, supporting vascular health and enhancing blood flow, which can boost libido.

3. Green Elixir
    - 1 cup spinach
    - 1 green apple
    - 1/2 cucumber
    - 1/2 lemon, peeled
    - A handful of mint

This green juice is loaded with magnesium to reduce stress and improve mood. The refreshing taste of mint and lemon adds to the invigorating properties of the juice.

4. Spiced Sunrise
    - 1 large carrot
    - 1/2 sweet potato, peeled
    - 1/2 inch turmeric or ginger root
    - 1/4 teaspoon cinnamon

Both carrots and sweet potatoes are high in Vitamin A and antioxidants, which are vital for hormone synthesis and libido enhancement. Turmeric and cinnamon help in reducing inflammation and improving heart health.

5. Avocado Love Smoothie
  - 1 ripe avocado
  - 1 banana
  - 1 cup coconut water
  - 1 tablespoon honey or to taste

Avocado is rich in potassium and heart-healthy fats that are essential for hormone production and libido. Banana adds a creamy texture and extra potassium.

Usage and Benefits
These juices are best consumed fresh, ideally in the morning or early afternoon to maximize their energizing effects. Regular consumption can lead to improved energy

levels, better circulation, enhanced mood, and a noticeable boost in libido.

By integrating these supercharged juices into your daily diet, you not only enhance your libido but also contribute to your overall health. These nutrient-packed beverages provide a natural, delicious way to boost your sexual health and energy levels.

Juices to Enhance Blood Flow and Circulation

When it comes to boosting libido and enhancing sexual health, the role of nutrition cannot be overstated. Supercharged juices, packed with specific nutrients, can significantly improve blood flow and circulation, which are crucial for sexual performance and overall vitality. In this detailed exploration, we will delve into how certain juices can be used to enhance libido by focusing on key ingredients that stimulate blood flow and improve cardiovascular health.

- Key Ingredients for Libido-Boosting Juices

1. Beets: Beets are rich in nitrates, which the body converts into nitric oxide. Nitric oxide helps dilate blood vessels, improving blood flow to all parts of the body, including the genital area. This can enhance erectile function and overall sexual arousal.

2. Watermelon: This fruit contains citrulline, an amino acid that may increase nitric oxide levels in the body. Like beets, this has the effect of relaxing blood vessels and increasing blood flow, which can enhance sexual stamina and performance.

3. Pomegranate: Studies have shown that pomegranate juice can lower blood pressure and improve blood flow. Pomegranate is also rich in antioxidants, which protect the nitric oxide in the body from being destroyed by free radicals.

4. Ginger: Ginger is another powerful circulation booster. It works by expanding the blood vessels and increasing body heat, which in turn helps blood flow more freely, enhancing sexual sensation and pleasure.

5. Garlic: While not traditionally used in juices, garlic can be a potent addition to them. Garlic contains allicin, which can improve blood flow and increase blood vessel flexibility. Small amounts can be juiced with other veggies to mask the strong flavor.

6. Leafy Greens: Spinach, kale, and other leafy greens are high in nitrates, much like beets. They are also loaded with

antioxidants, vitamins, and minerals that promote overall health and support vascular health.

- Creating Your Libido-Enhancing Juice

To make a supercharged juice for improving libido, consider a combination that includes several of the ingredients listed above. For example, a potent juice might consist of beetroot, a slice of watermelon, a handful of pomegranate seeds, a small piece of ginger, and a leafy green like spinach. This combination not only enhances blood flow but also improves stamina and can help maintain energy levels.

- Juicing Tips

- Use Fresh Ingredients: Always use fresh fruits and vegetables to maximize the nutritional benefits and flavor of your juices.
- Organic Produce: Choose organic when possible to avoid pesticides and chemicals

that can affect hormonal balance and overall health.
- Proper Hydration: Remember that hydration is key for overall vascular health, so include hydrating ingredients and drink plenty of water throughout the day.
- Consistency is Key: Regular consumption of these juices can help maintain their benefits, so include them as part of your daily routine.

- Health Considerations

While these juices are natural and generally considered safe, it's important to consume them as part of a balanced diet. People with certain medical conditions, such as kidney stones or gastroesophageal reflux disease, should exercise caution, particularly with beet and citrus juices. Always consult with a healthcare provider if you're unsure about introducing a new element into your diet, especially if you are on medication or have a chronic health condition.

Supercharged juices are a delicious and natural way to enhance libido and improve sexual health by boosting blood flow and circulation. By incorporating these juices into your daily routine, you can enjoy the dual benefits of increased sexual vitality and improved overall wellness. Whether it's a refreshing start to your day or a sweet way to end your meals, these juices could be the boost your body needs to perform at its best, both in and out of the bedroom.

Chapter 4: Juicing for Hormonal Balance

Understanding Hormonal Influences on Libido

Hormonal balance is crucial for maintaining overall health and well-being, including sexual health and libido. The endocrine system, which regulates hormones, influences everything from mood and energy levels to sexual function and libido. Hormonal imbalances can result in various symptoms, including fluctuations in sexual desire. Juicing, as part of a balanced diet, can be a natural and effective way to support hormonal balance and potentially boost libido.

Understanding Hormones and Libido

Libido, or sexual desire, is largely influenced by hormones such as estrogen, testosterone, and progesterone. In women, estrogen and progesterone play significant roles in sexual function, affecting everything from sexual desire to vaginal lubrication. In men, testosterone is the key hormone influencing libido. An imbalance in any of these hormones can lead to decreased libido and other sexual health issues.

The Role of Nutrition in Hormonal Balance

Nutrition plays a pivotal role in supporting the endocrine system. Vitamins, minerals, and antioxidants found in fruits and vegetables help to detoxify the body and support the production and regulation of hormones. Juicing is an excellent way to consume a concentrated amount of these nutrients, which can aid in enhancing overall hormonal balance.

Effective Ingredients for Juicing

1. Cruciferous Vegetables - Broccoli, kale, cauliflower, and Brussels sprouts are rich in indole-3-carbinol, which helps in detoxifying excess estrogen from the body. This is particularly beneficial for women with estrogen dominance, a condition that can suppress libido.

2. Citrus Fruits - Rich in vitamin C, citrus fruits like oranges, grapefruits, and lemons help improve overall immune function and assist in reducing cortisol levels. Elevated cortisol can negatively impact sex hormones.

3. Beets - High in the mineral boron, which is associated with the production of sexual hormones. Beets also help increase blood flow, which can enhance libido.

4. Ginger - Known for its anti-inflammatory properties, ginger can improve circulation and enhance blood flow, important for sexual function.

5. Pomegranate - Studies suggest that pomegranate juice can increase testosterone levels in both men and women, potentially boosting sexual desire and mood.

6. Leafy Greens - Spinach, chard, and other leafy greens are high in magnesium, a mineral that supports the production of sex hormones.

Juicing Recipes for Hormonal Balance

1. Green Detoxifier
    - 2 cups kale
    - 1 cup spinach
    - 1/2 green apple
    - 1/2 lemon, peeled
    - 1-inch piece of ginger

 This juice helps detoxify the liver, which is crucial for regulating hormones.

2. Beet Bliss

- 1 large beet
- 1 apple
- 1 carrot
- 1-inch piece of ginger

This blend not only supports hormonal health but also improves circulation, enhancing libido.

3. Citrus Burst
  - 2 oranges
  - 1/2 grapefruit
  - 1/2 lemon

 This vitamin C-rich juice helps lower cortisol levels and supports overall hormonal balance.

Juicing for hormonal balance is about more than just improving libido. It encompasses a holistic approach to nourishing the body and supporting the endocrine system. A well-planned juicing regimen, combined with a balanced diet and healthy lifestyle, can contribute significantly to hormonal health, impacting libido and overall vitality positively. Always consult with a healthcare provider before starting any new dietary regimen, especially if you have underlying health conditions or are on medication.

Hormone-Balancing Ingredients and Recipes

Juicing for hormonal balance involves incorporating specific fruits, vegetables, and herbs into your diet that are known for their potential to regulate hormonal levels. This approach can be especially helpful for addressing hormonal imbalances that affect mood, metabolism, fertility, and overall health. Here, we explore key hormone-balancing ingredients and provide recipes to integrate these into a balanced diet.

Hormone-Balancing Ingredients:

1. Cruciferous Vegetables:
   - Examples: Broccoli, cauliflower, kale, and Brussels sprouts.
   - Benefits: These vegetables contain indole-3-carbinol, which is converted in the body to a compound known as DIM (diindolylmethane). DIM helps to balance estrogen levels and has been shown to promote a healthy balance of good versus potentially harmful estrogen metabolites.

2. Leafy Greens:
   - Examples: Spinach, Swiss chard, and collard greens.
   - Benefits: Rich in magnesium, which plays a crucial role in hormone regulation. Magnesium can help with PMS symptoms and support thyroid function.

3. Berries:

 - Examples: Blueberries, strawberries, and raspberries.
 - Benefits: High in antioxidants, which protect cells from damage, including cells that produce hormones. They also help reduce inflammation and can help manage hormone-driven mood swings.

4. Citrus Fruits:
 - Examples: Lemons, oranges, and grapefruit.
 - Benefits: They are high in vitamin C, which is essential for adrenal gland function. The adrenal glands play a significant role in hormone production, including the stress hormones cortisol and adrenaline.

5. Avocado:
 - Benefits: Rich in beta-sitosterol, which can help balance the stress hormone cortisol. Avocados are also high in monounsaturated fat, which is critical for reproductive hormone production.

6. Seeds:
   - Examples: Flax seeds, chia seeds, and pumpkin seeds.
   - Benefits: Flax seeds are particularly known for their lignans, which can help balance estrogen levels. Pumpkin seeds are rich in zinc, vital for testosterone and progesterone production.

7. Beets:
   - Benefits: High in nitrates that improve blood flow and can help lower blood pressure. Beets also contain betaine, which supports liver function and helps the body eliminate excess hormones.

8. Herbs:
   - Examples: Maca, ashwagandha, and turmeric.
   - Benefits: Maca root is known for its ability to enhance fertility and balance hormone levels. Ashwagandha supports thyroid function and helps regulate cortisol

levels. Turmeric, with its active ingredient curcumin, has potent anti-inflammatory properties and can aid in hormone balance.

Juicing Recipes for Hormonal Balance:

1. Green Detox Juice:
   - Ingredients: 1 cup kale, ½ cup spinach, 1 green apple, ½ cucumber, 1 celery stalk, juice of ½ lemon.
   - Benefits: Detoxifies the body and supports liver health, essential for hormone balance.

2. Berry Citrus Boost:
   - Ingredients: 1 cup mixed berries, 1 orange, ½ grapefruit, 1 carrot.
   - Benefits: Boosts antioxidant intake and supports adrenal health.

3. Anti-Inflammatory Juice:
   - Ingredients: ½ beet, 1 inch turmeric root, 1 inch ginger root, 1 carrot, 1 apple.

- Benefits: Reduces inflammation and supports liver detoxification.

4. Seed Power Juice:
   - Ingredients: 1 apple, 1 pear, 1 tablespoon ground flax seeds, 1 tablespoon chia seeds, juice of 1 lemon.
   - Benefits: Balances estrogen and promotes digestive health.

When using juicing as a tool for hormonal balance, it's important to maintain a balanced diet and consult healthcare professionals, especially for those with thyroid issues or other hormonal disorders. Juicing can be a powerful complement to lifestyle changes, medication, and other dietary adjustments aimed at achieving hormonal equilibrium.

Managing Stress and Cortisol Levels through Juicing

Juicing for hormonal balance, particularly in the management of stress and cortisol levels, offers a natural and holistic approach to improving overall health and well-being. When our hormones are out of balance, especially stress hormones like cortisol, it can lead to various health issues, including fatigue, weight gain, and mood disturbances. Juicing can play a crucial role in helping regulate these hormones by providing the body with a concentrated source of nutrients that support hormonal health.

Understanding Cortisol and Its Effects

Cortisol, often referred to as the stress hormone, is produced by the adrenal glands in response to stress and low blood glucose concentration. While cortisol is vital for various bodily functions, including regulating metabolism and immune response, chronic elevated cortisol levels can lead to several health problems. These include suppressed immunity, hypertension, high blood sugar, insulin resistance, carbohydrate cravings, metabolic syndrome, and increased abdominal fat.

- Key Nutrients and Their Roles

Several nutrients are particularly important for managing cortisol levels and enhancing hormonal balance:

1. Vitamin C - Found in high levels in citrus fruits, bell peppers, and dark leafy greens, vitamin C has been shown to help reduce cortisol levels and improve the body's response to stress.

2. Magnesium - Often referred to as the relaxation mineral, magnesium can be found in spinach, chard, and pumpkin seeds. It helps to calm the nervous system and is essential for hundreds of biochemical reactions in the body, including those that help regulate cortisol levels.

3. B Vitamins - These are crucial for energy production and the proper function of the nervous system. B vitamins can help improve mood and reduce stress, leading to lower cortisol levels. Good sources include leafy greens, beets, and avocados.

4. Omega-3 Fatty Acids - While not typically found in juice, adding a splash of flaxseed oil or chia seeds to your juice can provide omega-3s, which are known to reduce inflammation and help manage stress levels.

5. Antioxidants - Fruits and vegetables like blueberries, apples, and carrots are high in

antioxidants, which combat oxidative stress, a by-product of high cortisol levels.

- Effective Juicing Recipes for Hormonal Balance

1. Green Goodness - Spinach, kale, cucumber, green apple, celery, and lemon. This juice is rich in magnesium, vitamin C, and B vitamins.

2. Citrus Bliss - Oranges, grapefruit, lemon, and a hint of mint. This refreshing mix boosts vitamin C to help regulate cortisol levels.

3. Berry Boost - Blueberries, strawberries, raspberries, and a small beet. Berries and beets are high in antioxidants and natural nitrates, which improve blood flow and reduce stress.

4. Tropical Calm - Pineapple, mango, and coconut water. Pineapple contains

bromelain, an enzyme that can help improve digestion and reduce inflammation.

- Tips for Juicing

- Always use fresh, organic produce to minimize exposure to pesticides.
- Drink juice on an empty stomach to maximize nutrient absorption.
- Avoid adding too many fruits to prevent excessive sugar intake.
- Drink freshly made juice immediately to benefit from the full nutrient content.

Incorporating juicing into your daily routine can be a powerful way to support hormonal balance and manage stress and cortisol levels. By selecting the right ingredients, you can harness the natural healing power of fruits and vegetables to improve your health and resilience against stress. Remember, while juicing can be a beneficial addition to a balanced diet, it should be part of a comprehensive approach to health that includes other lifestyle factors such as regular exercise, adequate sleep, and stress management techniques.

Chapter 5: Supporting Sexual Health Naturally

Detoxifying Juices for a Healthy Body and Mind

Maintaining optimal sexual health is essential for overall well-being. However, many individuals may struggle with issues related to sexual health due to factors such as poor diet, sedentary lifestyle, stress, and environmental toxins. Fortunately, there are natural ways to support sexual health, and one powerful method is through the consumption of detoxifying juices.

Supporting Sexual Health Naturally: Detoxifying Juices for a Healthy Body and Mind explores the intersection between nutrition, detoxification, and sexual wellness. In this comprehensive guide, readers will discover how incorporating fresh, nutrient-rich juices into their daily routine can help cleanse the body, boost vitality, and enhance sexual function.

It delves into common issues that may impact sexual function, such as hormonal imbalances, inflammation, and oxidative stress, and explains how detoxifying juices can help address these underlying factors.

Each chapter explores a different aspect of sexual health and offers delicious juice recipes specifically designed to target those areas. From hormone-balancing blends to antioxidant-rich concoctions, readers will find a variety of recipes tailored to support libido, stamina, fertility, and overall sexual vitality.

Furthermore, the book goes beyond just recipes by providing in-depth information on the nutritional benefits of each ingredient used in the juices. Readers will learn about the specific vitamins, minerals, antioxidants, and phytonutrients found in fruits, vegetables, and herbs that contribute to sexual health and well-being.

Moreover, the book emphasizes the importance of holistic health by discussing lifestyle factors that can impact sexual function, such as exercise, stress management, and adequate sleep. It offers practical tips and strategies for incorporating these practices into daily life to promote a balanced and fulfilling sex life.

Supporting Sexual Health Naturally also addresses common misconceptions and myths surrounding sexual health and detoxification, providing evidence-based information to empower readers to make informed choices about their health.

Overall, this book serves as a comprehensive resource for anyone looking to optimize their sexual health naturally. Whether you're struggling with specific sexual health issues or simply want to enhance your overall well-being, the detoxifying juices and lifestyle strategies outlined in this guide offer a holistic approach to supporting sexual vitality and achieving a healthy body and mind.

By embracing the power of nature's healing ingredients and adopting a holistic approach to wellness, readers can embark on a journey towards improved sexual health, vitality, and fulfillment. Supporting Sexual Health Naturally is not just a book—it's a roadmap to a healthier, happier, and more vibrant life.

Recipes for Immune System Support and Overall Wellbeing

Maintaining optimal sexual health is essential for overall well being however, with the abundance of processed foods and lifestyle stressors, many individuals struggle to prioritize their sexual health. This note aims to provide valuable insights and guidance on supporting sexual health naturally through wholesome recipes designed to boost the immune system and promote overall wellness.

Understanding the importance of sexual health goes beyond physical intimacy; it encompasses emotional, mental, and social wellbeing. Supporting sexual health requires a holistic approach that addresses various factors, including nutrition, exercise, stress management, and sleep hygiene.

The Role of Nutrition in Sexual Health: Nutrition plays a crucial role in supporting sexual health by providing essential nutrients that fuel the body and promote hormonal balance. Incorporating nutrient-rich foods into your diet can enhance libido, improve sexual function, and boost overall vitality. The recipes included in this book are carefully crafted to harness the power of natural ingredients known for their aphrodisiac properties and immune-boosting benefits.

Recipes for Immune System Support:
A strong immune system is vital for maintaining sexual health and overall wellbeing. The recipes in this book focus on incorporating immune-boosting ingredients such as fruits, vegetables, herbs, and spices rich in antioxidants, vitamins, and minerals. From vibrant smoothie bowls to nourishing soups and hearty salads, each recipe is designed to support immune function and enhance vitality.

Aphrodisiac Foods and Their Benefits:
Certain foods have been revered for their aphrodisiac properties for centuries, believed to enhance sexual desire, arousal, and performance. This book explores the science behind these aphrodisiac foods and

how they can positively impact sexual health. From decadent dark chocolate desserts to tantalizing seafood dishes and aromatic herbal teas, each recipe celebrates the sensual pleasures of food while nourishing the body and soul.

Stress Management and Sexual Health:
Chronic stress can negatively impact sexual health by affecting hormone levels, libido, and overall vitality. Incorporating stress-reducing practices such as meditation, yoga, and mindfulness can help promote relaxation and enhance sexual wellbeing. The recipes in this book are complemented by tips for managing stress and fostering a sense of calm and balance in daily life.

Sleep and Sexual Health:
Quality sleep is essential for sexual health and overall wellness. Poor sleep can disrupt hormone balance, reduce libido, and impair sexual function. This book provides recipes

designed to support restful sleep, incorporating ingredients known for their calming and sleep-promoting properties. From soothing herbal teas to nourishing bedtime snacks, each recipe aims to enhance sleep quality and rejuvenate the body.

Supporting sexual health naturally is a journey that begins with nourishing the body, mind, and spirit. By incorporating nutrient-rich foods, stress-reducing practices, and restorative sleep habits into your lifestyle, you can enhance sexual vitality, boost immune function, and cultivate overall wellbeing. The recipes and insights shared in this book are intended to inspire and empower you on your path to optimal sexual health and vitality.

Juices for Improving Sleep Quality and Restoring Vitality

Maintaining sexual health and vitality these days are essential for overall well-being and quality of life. Yet, many individuals struggle with issues such as low libido, erectile dysfunction, and decreased sexual satisfaction, often due to factors like stress, poor sleep quality, and inadequate nutrition.

This note aims to provide valuable insights into how natural remedies, particularly juices made from fresh fruits and vegetables, can support sexual health by improving sleep quality and restoring vitality. By harnessing the power of nature's bounty, individuals can enhance their sexual vitality, rejuvenate their bodies, and experience greater satisfaction in their intimate relationships.

Understanding the Link Between Sleep Quality and Sexual Health

Quality sleep is paramount for maintaining optimal sexual health and function. During sleep, the body undergoes essential processes such as hormone regulation, tissue repair, and rejuvenation, all of which contribute to overall well-being, including sexual vitality. Conversely, poor sleep quality can disrupt hormonal balance, increase stress levels, and diminish libido and sexual performance.

The Role of Nutrition in Sexual Health

Nutrition plays a crucial role in supporting sexual health by providing the body with essential nutrients and antioxidants that promote hormonal balance, improve circulation, and enhance overall vitality. Fruits and vegetables, in particular, are rich sources of vitamins, minerals, and phytonutrients that have been shown to benefit sexual function and libido.

The Power of Juicing for Sexual Health

Juicing offers a convenient and efficient way to incorporate a variety of nutrient-dense fruits and vegetables into the diet, providing a potent boost to sexual health and vitality. By extracting the natural juices from fresh produce, individuals can concentrate essential nutrients and antioxidants into a delicious and easily digestible form, promoting optimal health from within.

Key Ingredients for Sexual Health Juices

Several fruits and vegetables are renowned for their aphrodisiac properties and ability to support sexual health. Ingredients such as watermelon, pomegranate, beets, spinach, and ginger are rich in vitamins, minerals, and bioactive compounds that promote blood flow, enhance stamina, and increase libido.

Recipes for Sexual Health Juices

- *Passion Pomegranate Elixir*: A tantalizing blend of fresh pomegranate seeds, watermelon, and ginger, this juice is bursting with antioxidants and nutrients that promote blood flow and boost libido.

- *Vitality Beet Booster*: Rich in nitrates and iron, this juice combines beets, carrots, and spinach to support circulation, increase energy levels, and enhance sexual stamina.

- *Sensual Green Goddess*: A revitalizing mix of kale, cucumber, celery, and green apple, this juice provides a potent dose of vitamins and minerals that promote hormonal balance and overall vitality.

Incorporating Sexual Health Juices into Your Routine

Adding sexual health juices to your daily routine is simple and effortless. Enjoy them as a refreshing beverage in the morning, as a midday pick-me-up, or as a prelude to intimate moments with your partner. Experiment with different combinations of fruits and vegetables to find the flavors and ingredients that resonate with you.

By embracing natural remedies such as sexual health juices, individuals can take proactive steps towards improving sleep quality, restoring vitality, and enhancing sexual satisfaction. With the power of nature's bounty at their fingertips, they can nourish their bodies, rejuvenate their minds, and cultivate a deeper connection with their sexual selves. Let these juices be a delicious and invigorating addition to your journey towards optimal sexual health and vitality.

Chapter 6: Lifestyle Tips for Optimal Sexual Wellness

Exercise and Movement: Enhancing Your Libido Naturally

Sexual wellness is an integral part of overall health and happiness, and incorporating regular exercise and movement into your lifestyle can play a significant role in enhancing your libido and sexual satisfaction naturally. In this note, we'll explore the importance of exercise and movement for sexual wellness, as well as provide practical tips for incorporating physical activity into your daily routine.

Understanding the Connection Between Exercise and Libido

Regular exercise has been shown to have numerous benefits for sexual health and function. Physical activity increases blood flow throughout the body, including to the genitals, which can enhance arousal and sexual responsiveness. Additionally, exercise releases endorphins and other feel-good hormones, reducing stress and anxiety levels, which are common barriers to sexual desire.

Types of Exercise for Sexual Wellness

1. Cardiovascular Exercise: Activities such as walking, running, swimming, and cycling are excellent forms of cardiovascular exercise that can improve circulation, boost stamina, and increase overall energy levels, all of which can contribute to a more satisfying sex life.

2. Strength Training: Building muscle strength and endurance through activities like weightlifting and bodyweight exercises not only improves physical fitness but also enhances confidence and body image, leading to greater sexual self-esteem.

3. Yoga and Pilates: These mind-body practices focus on flexibility, balance, and mindfulness, promoting relaxation and reducing tension in both the body and mind. Yoga, in particular, includes poses specifically designed to increase blood flow to the pelvic area and improve sexual function.

4. Pelvic Floor Exercises: Strengthening the pelvic floor muscles through exercises like Kegels can enhance sexual sensation, improve bladder control, and help prevent erectile dysfunction and other sexual health issues.

Incorporating Exercise into Your Routine

1. Set Realistic Goals: Start by setting achievable fitness goals based on your current level of fitness and lifestyle. Gradually increase the intensity and

duration of your workouts as your stamina and strength improve.

2. Find Activities You Enjoy: Experiment with different types of exercise to find activities that you genuinely enjoy. Whether it's dancing, hiking, or playing a sport, incorporating fun and enjoyable activities into your routine can make exercise feel less like a chore and more like a rewarding experience.

3. Make It Social: Exercise with a partner or friend can make workouts more enjoyable and motivate you to stay consistent. Consider joining a sports team, fitness class, or exercise group to connect with others who share your interests.

4. Schedule Regular Exercise Sessions: Treat exercise as an essential part of your self-care routine by scheduling regular workout sessions into your calendar. Aim for at least 150 minutes of moderate-intensity aerobic

activity or 75 minutes of vigorous-intensity activity per week, along with muscle-strengthening exercises on two or more days.

5. Be Mindful of Your Body: Listen to your body's signals and avoid overexertion or pushing yourself too hard, especially if you're new to exercise or recovering from an injury. Pay attention to how different types of exercise affect your energy levels and mood, and adjust your routine accordingly.

Incorporating regular exercise and movement into your lifestyle is a powerful way to enhance your libido, improve sexual function, and promote overall sexual wellness. By prioritizing physical activity and making it a consistent part of your routine, you can enjoy the numerous benefits that exercise has to offer for both your physical and emotional well-being. Remember that every step you take towards improving your fitness is a step towards a healthier and more fulfilling sex life.

Stress Management Techniques for a Healthy Mind and Body

Sexual wellness is an integral aspect of overall well-being, encompassing physical, mental, and emotional health. In today's fast-paced world, stress has become a common factor that can significantly impact sexual health and satisfaction. This note aims to provide comprehensive lifestyle tips and stress management techniques to promote optimal sexual wellness and support a healthy mind and body.

Understanding Stress and Sexual Wellness

Stress is a natural response to various life challenges, but chronic stress can have detrimental effects on sexual health. High levels of stress can lead to decreased libido, erectile dysfunction, and difficulty reaching orgasm, among other issues. Additionally, stress can negatively impact relationships, communication, and intimacy between partners.

Lifestyle Tips for Promoting Sexual Wellness

1. Prioritize Self-Care: Engage in regular self-care practices such as adequate sleep, nutritious diet, regular exercise, and relaxation techniques. Taking care of your physical and mental health is essential for overall well-being, including sexual health.

2. Manage Stress Effectively: Identify sources of stress in your life and develop strategies to manage them effectively. This may include practicing mindfulness

meditation, deep breathing exercises, progressive muscle relaxation, or yoga. Find activities that help you relax and unwind, promoting a calm and peaceful state of mind.

3. Maintain a Healthy Lifestyle: Adopting a healthy lifestyle can positively impact sexual wellness. Limit alcohol consumption, avoid smoking, and practice safe sex to reduce the risk of sexually transmitted infections. Eat a balanced diet rich in fruits, vegetables, lean proteins, and whole grains to support overall health and vitality.

4. Communicate Openly with Your Partner: Effective communication is key to a healthy and satisfying sexual relationship. Discuss your desires, concerns, and boundaries with your partner openly and honestly. Mutual understanding and respect are essential for fostering intimacy and connection in a relationship.

5. Explore Sensuality and Intimacy: Focus on enhancing sensuality and intimacy with your partner through non-sexual activities such as cuddling, kissing, and intimate conversations. Building emotional closeness and connection can deepen intimacy and strengthen the bond between partners.

6. Seek Professional Help When Needed: If stress or other factors are significantly impacting your sexual wellness, don't hesitate to seek support from a healthcare provider or mental health professional. They can offer guidance, support, and resources to address underlying issues and improve sexual health.

Optimal sexual wellness is achievable through a combination of lifestyle factors, stress management techniques, and open communication with your partner. By prioritizing self-care, managing stress effectively, and fostering intimacy and connection, individuals can promote a healthy mind and body, leading to enhanced sexual satisfaction and overall well-being. Remember that sexual wellness is an essential component of a fulfilling and balanced life, deserving of attention, care, and nurturing.

The Importance of Communication and Intimacy in Relationships

Maintaining sexual wellness is crucial for overall well-being and relationship satisfaction. This note serves as a comprehensive guide to lifestyle tips aimed at promoting optimal sexual health, with a particular focus on fostering communication and intimacy within relationships.

Sexual wellness encompasses physical, emotional, mental, and social aspects of sexuality. It involves feeling positively about one's body, having satisfying sexual experiences, and fostering healthy relationships built on trust and respect. Achieving sexual wellness requires a holistic approach that addresses both individual and relational factors.

The Role of Communication

Effective communication is the cornerstone of healthy sexual relationships. Open and honest dialogue allows partners to express their desires, boundaries, and concerns, fostering mutual understanding and trust. Communication also enables couples to explore new sexual experiences, negotiate consent, and navigate challenges together.

Tips for Enhancing Communication:

1. Create a Safe Space: Establish an environment where both partners feel comfortable discussing sexual topics without fear of judgment or criticism.

2. Practice Active Listening: Listen attentively to your partner's needs and desires, validating their feelings and experiences.

3. Be Honest and Transparent: Share your own thoughts, feelings, and concerns openly, promoting transparency and authenticity in the relationship.

4. Use I Statements: Communicate using I statements to express your own feelings and experiences without blaming or accusing your partner.

5. Seek Professional Help: If communication barriers persist, consider seeking guidance from a therapist or counselor specializing in sexual health and relationships.

The Power of Intimacy

Intimacy goes beyond physical attraction and sexual activity; it involves emotional closeness, vulnerability, and connection between partners. Cultivating intimacy strengthens the bond between couples, enhancing relationship satisfaction and sexual fulfillment. Intimate relationships are characterized by trust, empathy, and mutual support, fostering a sense of security and belonging.

Tips for Fostering Intimacy:

1. Prioritize Quality Time Together: Dedicate time to connect with your partner through shared activities, meaningful conversations, and affectionate gestures.
2. Express Gratitude and Appreciation: Acknowledge and celebrate your partner's strengths, efforts, and contributions to the relationship, fostering a sense of mutual admiration and respect.
3. Practice Physical Affection: Engage in non-sexual touch, such as cuddling, holding

hands, and hugging, to promote feelings of closeness and connection.

4. Embrace Vulnerability: Share your innermost thoughts, fears, and dreams with your partner, allowing them to see your authentic self and vice versa.

5. Explore Shared Interests: Discover new hobbies, interests, and experiences together, deepening your connection and creating lasting memories.

By prioritizing communication and intimacy in their relationships, individuals can enhance their sexual wellness and overall relationship satisfaction. Through open dialogue, mutual respect, and emotional connection, couples can navigate challenges, celebrate successes, and cultivate fulfilling and satisfying sexual experiences together. Remember that sexual wellness is an ongoing journey that requires effort, commitment, and dedication from both partners.

Chapter 7: Integrating Juicing with Traditional Medicine

Exploring the Intersection of Natural Remedies and Modern Medicine

Over the years, there has been a resurgence of interest in holistic approaches to health and wellness, with many individuals seeking out natural remedies to complement traditional medical treatments. One such approach that has gained popularity is juicing – the process of extracting the nutrient-rich juices from fruits and vegetables to create delicious and nutritious beverages.

This note delves into the intersection of juicing and traditional medicine, exploring how these two approaches can be integrated to promote overall health and well-being. By understanding the benefits of juicing and its potential synergies with modern medicine, individuals can make informed decisions about their health and explore new avenues for healing and self-care.

The Benefits of Juicing:
Juicing offers a convenient and delicious way to increase your intake of fruits and vegetables, which are rich in essential vitamins, minerals, and antioxidants. These nutrients play crucial roles in supporting the body's natural detoxification processes, boosting the immune system, and promoting overall health and vitality.

Also, juicing can help individuals maintain a healthy weight, improve digestion, and increase energy levels. By consuming fresh, nutrient-dense juices regularly, individuals may experience improvements in their skin, hair, and overall appearance, as well as enhanced mental clarity and focus.

Integration with Traditional Medicine:

While juicing is not a replacement for traditional medical treatments, it can complement existing therapies and support overall health and wellness. Many fruits and vegetables used in juicing have been studied for their potential health benefits, including their ability to reduce inflammation, lower blood pressure, and improve cardiovascular health.

By incorporating fresh juices into their diets, individuals can provide their bodies with the essential nutrients needed for optimal health and healing. Juicing can also be used as part of a holistic approach to managing chronic conditions such as diabetes, arthritis, and autoimmune disorders, alongside conventional medical treatments.

Exploring Synergies and Considerations: When integrating juicing with traditional medicine, it's essential to consider individual health needs, preferences, and any existing medical conditions. Consulting with a healthcare professional or nutritionist can help individuals develop personalized juicing plans that align with their overall health goals and medical treatment plans.

Additionally, it's important to recognize that while juicing can offer numerous health benefits, it's not suitable for everyone. Some individuals may need to limit their intake of certain fruits and vegetables due to allergies, sensitivities, or specific medical conditions. Moderation and variety are key when incorporating juices into a balanced diet.

Integrating juicing with traditional medicine offers an exciting opportunity to explore the synergies between natural remedies and modern healthcare practices. By incorporating fresh, nutrient-dense juices into their diets, individuals can support their overall health and well-being while complementing traditional medical treatments.

Ultimately, the key lies in finding a balance that works for each individual, taking into account their unique health needs, preferences, and lifestyle factors. Whether used as a daily wellness ritual or as part of a comprehensive treatment plan, juicing has the potential to enhance health, vitality, and longevity for those who embrace its benefits.

Collaborating with Healthcare Providers for Holistic Sexual Wellness

Over the years, the concept of holistic sexual wellness has gained traction as individuals seek comprehensive approaches to address sexual health issues beyond just medical treatments. Integrating juicing with traditional medicine offers a promising avenue for enhancing sexual well-being, as it combines the benefits of nutrient-rich juices with evidence-based medical interventions. This note explores the synergies between juicing and traditional medicine, emphasizing the importance of collaboration with healthcare providers for optimal outcomes.

- Benefits of Juicing for Sexual Wellness

- Nutrient Absorption: Juicing allows for the concentrated intake of essential vitamins, minerals, and antioxidants that support sexual health, including vitamin C, zinc, magnesium, and folate.

- Hydration: Proper hydration is essential for optimal sexual function, as it helps maintain blood flow and lubrication. Juices can contribute to hydration while providing additional nutrients beneficial for sexual wellness.

- Detoxification: Certain fruits and vegetables contain detoxifying properties that support liver function and hormone balance, which can positively impact sexual health.

- Alkalinity: Juices made from alkaline-rich foods, such as leafy greens and cucumbers, can help balance the body's pH levels, creating an environment conducive to sexual vitality.

Collaborating with Healthcare Providers

While juicing can offer valuable benefits for sexual wellness, it is essential to integrate this approach with traditional medicine under the guidance of healthcare providers. Collaboration with medical professionals, including primary care physicians, gynecologists, urologists, and nutritionists, ensures a comprehensive and evidence-based approach to sexual health.

- Key Considerations for Collaboration

- Medical History: Healthcare providers can assess individual medical histories, including underlying health conditions, medications, and allergies, to customize juicing recommendations and ensure compatibility with traditional treatments.

- Nutritional Needs: Nutritionists or dietitians can provide personalized guidance on juicing recipes and dietary modifications to address specific nutritional deficiencies or health goals related to sexual wellness.

- Monitoring and Evaluation: Regular monitoring of sexual health indicators, such as libido, erectile function, hormone levels, and overall well-being, allows healthcare providers to track progress and adjust treatment plans as needed.

- Education and Support: Healthcare providers play a crucial role in educating patients about the benefits and limitations of juicing for sexual wellness, as well as addressing any concerns or misconceptions. They can also offer emotional support and encouragement throughout the journey to better sexual health.

Integrating juicing with traditional medicine offers a holistic approach to sexual wellness that addresses the physical, emotional, and nutritional aspects of sexual health. By collaborating with healthcare providers, individuals can harness the synergies between juicing and conventional treatments to achieve optimal sexual well-being and enhance their overall quality of life.

Tips for Safe and Effective Integration of Juicing with Medication

Juicing has gained popularity as a method for enhancing health and wellness, offering a convenient way to consume a variety of fruits and vegetables in concentrated form. However, when it comes to integrating juicing with traditional medicine, particularly medication, it's essential to proceed with caution to ensure safety and effectiveness. This note provides valuable tips and considerations for individuals looking to incorporate juicing into their wellness routine while taking medication.

Understanding the Basics

Before delving into the integration of juicing with medication, it's crucial to have a solid understanding of both juicing and traditional medicine. Juicing involves the extraction of liquid from fruits and vegetables, typically using a juicer, to create nutrient-rich beverages. Traditional medicine encompasses a wide range of practices, including pharmaceutical medications prescribed by healthcare professionals to treat various health conditions.

Consultation with Healthcare Provider

One of the most important steps in integrating juicing with medication is consulting with a healthcare provider. Healthcare professionals, such as doctors or pharmacists, can provide personalized guidance based on an individual's medical history, current health status, and specific medication regimen. They can offer insights into potential interactions between certain fruits, vegetables, or supplements commonly used in juicing and prescribed medications.

Awareness of Potential Interactions

Certain fruits and vegetables commonly used in juicing may interact with specific medications, affecting their absorption, metabolism, or effectiveness. For example, grapefruit juice is known to interact with a wide range of medications, including statins, certain blood pressure medications, and immunosuppressants. Other fruits and vegetables, such as kale, spinach, and broccoli, contain compounds that may interfere with the metabolism of certain drugs.

Timing Considerations

The timing of juicing and medication intake is another crucial aspect to consider. Some medications may need to be taken on an empty stomach, while others should be taken with food to minimize side effects or enhance absorption. Individuals should consult their healthcare provider to determine the best timing for consuming juice in relation to their medication schedule.

Monitoring for Adverse Effects

When integrating juicing with medication, it's essential to monitor for any adverse effects or changes in health status. Individuals should pay attention to symptoms such as nausea, dizziness, changes in blood pressure or blood sugar levels, or any other unusual reactions that may occur after consuming juice alongside medication. Any concerning symptoms should be promptly reported to a healthcare provider for further evaluation.

Personalized Approach

It's important to recognize that the integration of juicing with medication is not a one-size-fits-all approach. Factors such as individual health goals, medical conditions, medication regimens, and dietary preferences should all be taken into account when developing a personalized plan for juicing alongside traditional medicine. Working closely with a healthcare provider can help individuals tailor their juicing practices to complement their overall wellness plan safely and effectively.

Integrating juicing with traditional medicine can be a valuable component of a holistic approach to health and wellness. By following the tips outlined in this note, individuals can navigate the integration process with confidence, ensuring that juicing enhances, rather than interferes with, their medication regimen. With careful consideration and guidance from healthcare professionals, individuals can reap the benefits of juicing while effectively managing their health conditions.

Conclusion

Embracing a Healthier, More Vibrant You:
Final Thoughts on Juicing for Sexual Health

In the exploration of integrating juicing with traditional medicine to enhance sexual health, it's imperative to recognize the holistic nature of well-being. Sexual health is not just about physical function; it encompasses emotional, mental, and relational aspects as well. Juicing can play a significant role in supporting overall health, which in turn can positively impact sexual vitality and satisfaction.

By nourishing the body with nutrient-dense juices, individuals can support circulation, hormone balance, and energy levels—all of which are crucial for optimal sexual function. Moreover, the abundance of vitamins, minerals, and antioxidants found in fresh fruits and vegetables can promote cardiovascular health, reduce inflammation, and support the body's natural detoxification processes, all of which contribute to enhanced sexual wellness.

It's essential to approach juicing for sexual health as part of a comprehensive lifestyle strategy that includes regular exercise, stress management, adequate sleep, and healthy relationships. Juicing can complement these lifestyle factors by providing a convenient and enjoyable way to increase intake of essential nutrients that support sexual vitality.

Furthermore, it's essential to consult with healthcare professionals, including naturopaths, nutritionists, and holistic practitioners, to ensure that juicing aligns with individual health goals and needs. Integrating juicing with traditional medicine can offer a synergistic approach to health and wellness, harnessing the power of both modern science and ancient wisdom to promote vitality and longevity.

Juicing for sexual health is not a quick fix or a standalone solution, but rather a valuable tool in the journey towards holistic well-being. By embracing juicing as part of a balanced and health-conscious lifestyle, individuals can unlock their full potential for vitality, pleasure, and fulfillment in all areas of life.

Resources for Further Exploration

- Books:
 - The Juicing Bible by Pat Crocker
 - Juicing for Health: 81 Juicing Recipes and 76 Ingredients Proven to Improve Health and Vitality by Mendocino Press
 - The Complete Guide to Juicing, Revised and Updated: Everything You Need to Know to Get the Most from Your Juicer by John Chatham

- Websites:
  - Juicing for Health (juicing-for-health.com)
  - Reboot with Joe (rebootwithjoe.com)
  - The Juicing Expert (thejuicingexpert.com)

- Online Communities:
  - Juicing for Health Facebook Group
  - Reddit Juicing Community (reddit.com/r/juicing)

- Podcasts:
  - The Juicing Podcast
  - The Ultimate Health Podcast

- Documentaries:
  - Fat, Sick & Nearly Dead (2010) - Directed by Joe Cross
  - Super Juice Me! (2014) - Directed by Jason Vale

- Professional Organizations:

- International Society for Sexual Medicine (issm.info)
- American Association of Sexuality Educators, Counselors, and Therapists (aasect.org)
- Integrative Medicine for Mental Health (immh.org)

These resources offer valuable information, inspiration, and support for those interested in exploring juicing for sexual health and overall well-being. Remember to approach any dietary or lifestyle changes with mindfulness and consideration for individual health needs, and always consult with qualified healthcare professionals for personalized guidance and advice.

Appendix: Recipe Index

Quick Reference Guide to Libido-Boosting Juice Recipes

Welcome to the Quick Reference Guide to Libido-Boosting Juice Recipes! In this comprehensive guide, you'll discover a variety of delicious and nutritious juice recipes designed to enhance your libido and improve your sexual vitality. Whether you're looking to spice up your love life or simply boost your overall well-being, these recipes offer a natural and enjoyable way to support your sexual health.

Each recipe in this guide is carefully crafted using a combination of fruits, vegetables, and other ingredients known for their libido-enhancing properties. From refreshing citrus blends to rich and decadent concoctions, there's something for everyone to enjoy. Plus, with easy-to-follow instructions and helpful tips, you'll be whipping up libido-boosting juices in no time.

But before we dive into the recipes, let's take a closer look at the ingredients featured in these juices and how they can help support a healthy libido:

1. Fruits: Fruits such as strawberries, watermelon, and figs are rich in vitamins, minerals, and antioxidants that can help improve blood flow and enhance sexual function.

2. Vegetables: Leafy greens like spinach and kale are packed with nutrients that support overall health and vitality, including magnesium and folate, which are important for sexual health.

3. Herbs and Spices: Ingredients like ginger, cinnamon, and ginseng have long been used in traditional medicine to boost libido and improve sexual performance.

4. Nuts and Seeds: Almonds, walnuts, and pumpkin seeds are excellent sources of essential fatty acids and zinc, which are important for hormone production and sexual health.

Now, without further ado, let's explore some tantalizing juice recipes that are sure to get your libido sizzling:

1. Passion Punch: This invigorating blend combines watermelon, strawberries, and mint for a refreshing burst of flavor that's perfect for a hot summer day.

2. Sensual Citrus: Oranges, grapefruits, and a hint of ginger come together in this zesty concoction that's sure to awaken your senses and revitalize your libido.

3. Exotic Elixir: Transport yourself to a tropical paradise with this exotic blend of pineapple, mango, and coconut water,

infused with a touch of turmeric for added spice.

4. Love Potion: Indulge in the decadent flavors of chocolate and cherries with this rich and creamy smoothie that's as delicious as it is libido-boosting.

5. Vitality Booster: Kick-start your day with this energizing blend of spinach, kale, and banana, packed with nutrients to fuel your body and enhance your sexual vitality.

Remember, the key to reaping the benefits of these libido-boosting juices is consistency. Incorporating them into your daily routine alongside a balanced diet and regular exercise can help support your sexual health and overall well-being over time.

Libido-Boosting Juice Recipes

1. Passion Potion: Pineapple, Mango, Ginger, and Lime

2. Berry Bliss: Blueberries, Raspberries, Strawberries, and Beetroot

3. Citrus Zest: Oranges, Grapefruits, and Lemons

4. Pomegranate Power: Pomegranate, Cherries, and Apple

5. Ginger Spice: Carrots, Apples, and Fresh Ginger

6. Watermelon Wonder: Watermelon, Cucumber, and Mint

7. Tropical Temptation: Papaya, Kiwi, and Pineapple

8. Green Goddess: Spinach, Kale, Apple, and Lemon

9. Beet Boost: Beets, Carrots, and Oranges

10. Mango Magic: Mango, Banana, and Coconut Water

11. Avocado Dream: Avocado, Pineapple, and Spinach

12. Spicy Citrus: Oranges, Grapefruits, Ginger, and Cayenne Pepper

13. Carrot Charm: Carrots, Oranges, and Ginger

14. Cucumber Cooler: Cucumber, Celery, Apple, and Mint

15. Lemon Lime Delight: Lemon, Lime, Honeydew Melon, and Mint

16. Melon Medley: Cantaloupe, Honeydew Melon, and Watermelon

17. Blueberry Blast: Blueberries, Banana, and Almond Milk

18. Cherry Cheer: Cherries, Spinach, and Pineapple

19. Peach Pleasure: Peaches, Mango, and Coconut Water

20. Apple Ambrosia: Apples, Grapes, and Cinnamons

21. Kiwi Kiss: Kiwi, Pineapple, and Spinach

22. Pineapple Paradise: Pineapple, Coconut Water, and Mint

23. Basil Berry Breeze: Strawberries, Blueberries, Basil, and Lime

24. Spinach Surprise: Spinach, Pear, Grapes, and Lemon

25. Grapefruit Glow: Grapefruits, Oranges, and Strawberries

26. Turmeric Tonic: Carrots, Oranges, Turmeric, and Ginger

27. Minty Marvel: Apples, Cucumbers, Mint, and Lemon

28. Guava Goddess: Guava, Mango, and Papaya

29. Passionate Pear: Pears, Strawberries, and Kiwi

30. Cinnamon Sensation: Apples, Cinnamon, and Honey

31. Lemon Ginger Elixir: Lemons, Ginger, Honey, and Water

32. Raspberry Rapture: Raspberries, Strawberries, and Blackberries

33. Carrot Apple Crush: Carrots, Apples, and Celery

34. Mango Mint Madness: Mango, Mint, Coconut Water, and Lime

35. Kale Kick: Kale, Pineapple, and Orange

36. Berry Basil Blast: Blueberries, Strawberries, Basil, and Coconut Water

37. Orange Carrot Splash: Oranges, Carrots, and Ginger

38. Pineapple Papaya Pleasure: Pineapple, Papaya, and Mango

These delicious and nutritious juice recipes are packed with libido-boosting ingredients to help spice up your love life and revitalize your energy levels. Enjoy these refreshing concoctions as part of a healthy lifestyle and reap the benefits of increased vitality and sexual wellness.

So why wait? Start exploring these delicious juice recipes today and take the first step towards reclaiming your sexual vitality and enhancing your love life.

Cheers 🥂 to a healthier, happier you!

www.ingramcontent.com/pod-product-compliance
Lightning Source LLC
Chambersburg PA
CBHW061647250726
48659CB00004B/1405